Acknowledgement

I0480555

The authors wish to extend their gratitude to a number of TB experts, public health officials/professionals, laboratory scientist, technicians and the Botswana National Tuberculosis Programme staff who contributed and helped with the development of this manuscript. The authors also wishes to thank their families, loved ones, colleagues and friends too many to mention here who provided ongoing support during the development of this project.

.

Table of Contents

Acronyms and Abbreviations

AIDS	Acquired Immunodeficiency Syndrome
BSL	Biosafety level
CDC	Centers for Disease Control and Prevention
CRI	Colorimetric Redox Indicator
DNA	Deoxyribonucleic Acid
DR-TB	Drug Resistant Tuberculosis
DST	Drug Susceptibility Testing
EMB	Ethambutol
FDA	Food and Drug Administration
FIND	Foundation for Innovative New Diagnostics
GC	Growth Control
HBC	High-Burden Countries
HIV	Human Immunodeficiency Virus
INH	Isoniazid
IUATLD	International Union Against Tuberculosis and Lung Disease
LJ	Löwenstein-Jensen

LJPM	Löwenstein-Jensen Proportion Method
LPA	Line Probe Assay
LRP	Luciferase Reporter Phages
MDR/RR-TB	Multidrug/Rifampicin Resistant Tuberculosis
MDR-TB	Multidrug - Resistant Tuberculosis
MGIT	Mycobacteria Growth Indicator Tube
MODS	Microscopic Observation Drug Susceptibility
MTB	Mycobacterium Tuberculosis
MTT	3-(4,5-dimethylthiazol-2-yl)-2,5-diphenyltetrazolium Bromide
NAAT	Nucleic Acid Amplification Test
NRA	Nitrate Reductase Assay
NTP	National Tuberculosis Programme
PNB	Para-Nitrobenzoic Acid
PCR	Polymerase Chain Reaction
PLWHA	People Living With HIV/AIDS
RIF	Rifampicin
RL/HBC	Resource Limited/High-Burden Countries
RLS	Resource Limited Settings

RR	Rifampicin Resistance
RR-TB	Rifampicin Resistant Tuberculosis
RT	Real-Time
SM	Streptomycin
SSA	Sub-Saharan Africa
TAT	Turnaround Time
TB	Tuberculosis
TDR	Research and Training in Tropical Diseases
TLA	Thin Layer Agar Method
USA	United States of America
UPS	Uninterrupted Power Supply
UV	Ultra-violet
WHO	World Health Organization
WRD	World Health Organization - Recommended Rapid Diagnostic
XDR-TB	Extensively Drug Resistant Tuberculosis

1. Introduction

Tuberculosis (TB) remains an important infectious disease and a major public health problem worldwide especially in the sub-Saharan African (SSA) Region. World Health Organization (WHO) estimates that one quarter of the world's population approximately 1.7 billion people are infected with *Mycobacteria tuberculosis* (MTB) the causative agent of TB [1,2]. This bacterial disease which most commonly affects the lungs is transmitted from person to person via droplets nuclei released into the air by coughing, sneezing, talking or singing from people with active respiratory disease. These droplets can remain in the air for several hours until they are removed by natural or mechanical ventilation. When a person inhales these droplets nuclei they can become infected with TB [1]. Congregate settings like health care facilities, prisons, refugee camps, rehabilitation centers, churches, military barracks, schools, markets, mines and factories are some of the potential areas for rapid transmission of the disease [1,3].

WHO estimates that 10 million (range, 9.0-11.1) incident cases of TB and 1.3 million deaths occurred worldwide in 2018 [1,4,5]. Geographically, most of the estimated number of TB cases occurred in the WHO region of South-East Asia (44%), the WHO African Region (24%), and the Western Pacific (18%) with smaller proportions of cases occurring in the Eastern Mediterranean Region (8.1%), the European Region (2.6%) and Region of the Americas (2.9%) [1]. Of the 10 million incident TB cases in 2018, eight countries accounted for two thirds of the global total: India (27%), China (9%), Indonesia (8%), the Phillipines (6%), Pakistan (6%), Nigeria (4%), Bangladesh (4%) and the Republic of South Africa (3%) [1]. However, the burden of the disease varied greatly among countries around the globe, from as few as 5 new cases per 100 000 population to more than 500 new cases per 100 000 population per year, with a global average of about 130.

There were under 10 incident cases per 100 000 population in most high-income countries, 150 - 400 cases per 100 000 population in most of the 30 high TB burden countries and above 500 cases per 100 000 population in TB endemic countries such as the Central African Republic, the Democratic People's Republic of Korea, Lesotho, Mozambique, Namibia, the Phillipines and the Republic of South Africa [1].

Many factors influence the progression from TB infection to disease, which is greatly dependent upon the strength of the body's cell-mediated immunity. Important factors include HIV infection, malnutrition, poverty, use of immunosuppressive drugs, alcoholism, bacillary load in the sputum, proximity of an individual to an infectious TB case, behavioural factors, tobacco smoke and many other socio-economic factors [6-8]. However, HIV infection remains the most powerful factor affecting disease progression [8].

Global efforts to manage and control the TB pandemic in recent years have been undermined by the emergence and spread of strains resistant to the most commonly used first-line anti-TB drugs: isoniazid (INH), rifampicin (RIF), streptomycin (SM), pyrazinamide (PZA) and ethambutol (EMB), and more specifically multidrug-resistant TB (MDR-TB) defined as resistance to at least INH and RIF- the two most powerful anti-TB drugs and rifampicin - resistant TB (RR-TB) defined as the in vitro resistance to RIF detected using phenotypic or genotypic methods, with or without resistance to other anti-TB drugs [1-3,9].

MDR/RR-TB is a serious global public health problem that threatens the significant progress made in TB care and prevention in recent decades [1,10]. The disease may result from a primary infection with a drug resistant strain of MTB or may develop during the course of patient therapy and usually as a product of inappropriate use of anti-TB drugs, either by the patient or by the practicing clinicians [11,12,14,15]. The latest anti-TB drug resistance surveillance data show that 3.4% of new TB cases and 18% of previously treated TB cases globally were estimated to have MDR/RR-TB in 2018. Recent WHO modelling of the incidence of MDR/RR-TB estimated that half a million (range, 417 000 - 556 000) new cases occurred in 2018 and MDR/RR-TB was responsible for approximately 214 000 (range, 133 000 - 295 000) deaths worldwide [1,2]. Three highly populated countries: India (27%), China (14%), and the Russian Federation (9%) accounted for about 50% of the global burden of the disease in 2018 [1,2].

Treatment of MDR/RR-TB is difficult and complicated as it requires second-line drugs such as aminoglycosides, fluoroquinolones, ethionamide, cycloserine, which are less effective, more toxic, some of which are only injectables, and more expensive than first-line agents [16-19]. Treatment duration is long, usually lasting between 9 months and up to 24 months supported by counselling and monitoring of adverse events [1,16,20]. However, recent data shows that outcomes for patients with MDR/RR-TB are generally poor with an estimated cure rate of only 50% - 60% compared with a 95% - 97% cure rate for patients with drug-susceptible strains of TB [1,11,16,18,21,22]. Recently new drugs such as bedaquiline and delamanid have been recommended for use by the WHO under specific conditions and may be added to a core of MDR/RR-TB regimen for improved patient outcomes [1,14].

The social and economic burden of MDR/RR-TB on patients and the health care system is self evident, given that it takes more than 20 months of daily therapy in most of the affected patients and the cost of treating an average MDR/RR-TB patient is 50 to 200 times higher than treating a drug susceptible TB case [23]. Thus to effectively address the threats of MDR/RR-TB, global initiatives are required to scale-up culture and drug susceptibility testing (DST) capacities, especially in high-burden countries (HBC) where such capacity is scarce. In parallel, efforts are also needed to expand the use of novel and emerging technologies (ie, molecular diagnostics) for the rapid determination of TB drug resistance [24]. Therefore, the purpose of this review is to describe laboratory-based diagnostic options currently available for testing MDR/RR-TB that can be used at different levels of the laboratory network to support patient management and global control of the disease. This review also aims to highlight key challenges associated with their implementation in low- and middle- income countries worldwide.

2. Global burden of MDR/RR-TB

The burden of DR-TB and in particular MDR/RR-TB is of major interest and concern at global, regional and country levels [1]. The Global Project on Anti-Tuberculosis Drug Resistance Surveillance of WHO (Global TB Project) and International Union Against Tuberculosis and Lung Disease (IUATLD) has been gathering data since 1994 in order to measure the prevalence of anti-TB drug resistance worldwide and to monitor the trend of the disease using standardized methodology [1]. Although the global magnitude of DR-TB remains unknown todate, national and regional studies and anecdotal evidence indicate that every region and country of the world has reported MDR/RR-TB [1,2]. Figure 1 shows the global coverage of drug-resistance surveillance data covering the period 1995 - 2019.

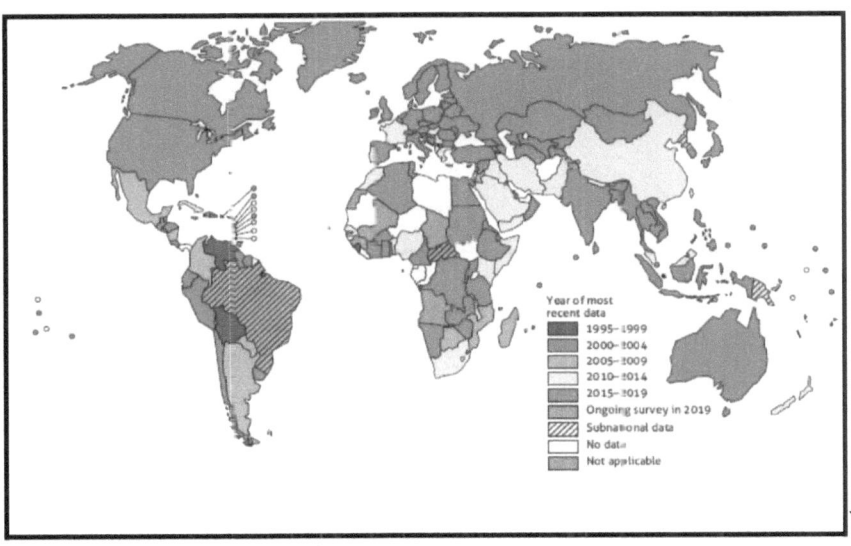

Figure 1: Global coverage of surveillance on drug resistance, 1995-2019

Source: WHO Global TB Report 2019

Globally in 2018, an estimated 3.4% of new TB cases and 18% of previously treated TB cases had MDR/RR-TB [1] (Table 1). It is also estimated that there were half a million new cases of RR-TB (of which 78% had MDR-TB) in 2018. The extent and burden of MDR/RR-TB varied significantly across countries and regions of the world surveyed [1,20,25], with the highest proportions of MDR/RR-TB reported in Eastern Europe. MDR/RR-TB in this region accounted for over 25% among new TB cases and above 50% among previously treated TB cases [1]. However, three most populous countries in the world together accounted for almost half of the total global MDR/RR-TB burden: India (27%), China (14%), and the Russian Federation (9%) [1]. Figure 2 and Figure 3 below shows the proportions of new and previously treated TB cases with MDR/RR-TB at country or territory level between 2004 and 2019.

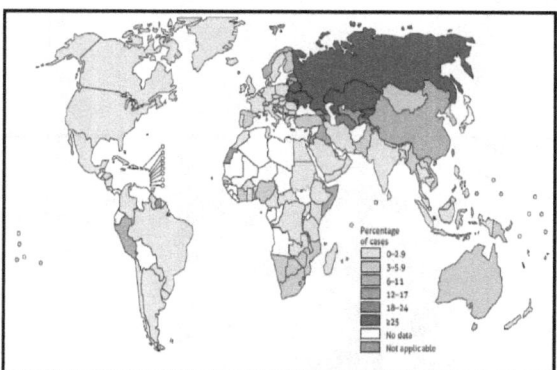

Figure 2: Percentage of new TB cases with MDR-TB/RR-TB; 2004-2019
Source: WHO Global TB Report 2019

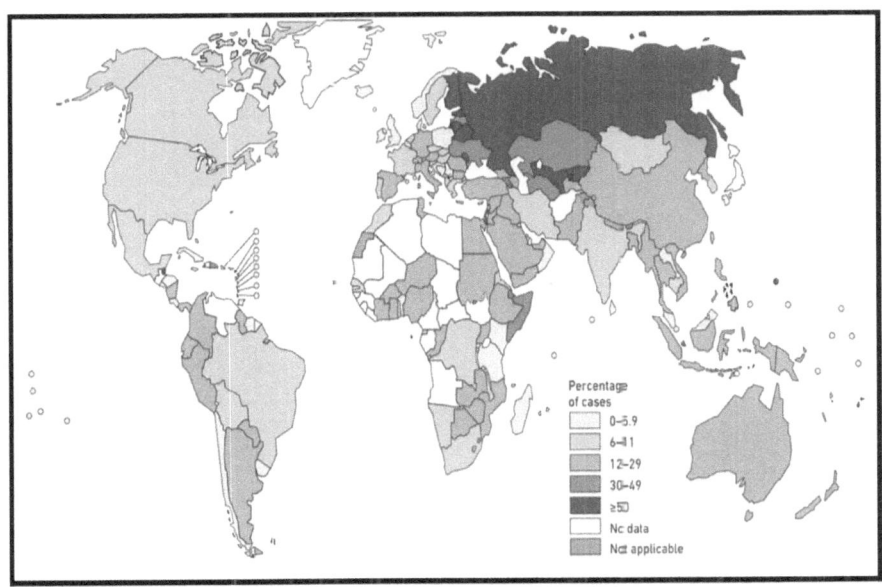

Figure 3: Percentage of previously treated TB cases with MDR/RR-TB; 2004 - 2019
Source: WHO Global TB Report 2019

2.1. The European epidemic

Most Western and Central European countries do not have a significant problem with drug resistance in newly diagnosed TB patients, reporting approximately 5-10% INH resistance and 1-2% MDR-TB. However, countries in Eastern Europe have reported significantly higher rates of MDR/RR-TB among new TB cases. These include Belarus (37%), Republic of Moldova (29%), Kyrgyzstan (29%), Kazakhstan (27%), Ukraine (29%), Uzbekistan (15%), the Russia Federation (35%), Tajikistan (21%) and Azerbaijan (12%) [1]. Table 1below shows the estimated incidence of MDR/RR-TB in 2018 by WHO Regions.

Table 1: Estimated Incidence of MDR/RR-TB in 2018 by WHO Regions				
WHO REGION	% of New TB cases with MDR/RR-TB	Range	% of Previously Treated TB Cases with MDR/RR-TB	Range
Africa	2.5	1.6 - 3.6	12	0.55 - 39
The Americas	2.5	1.5 - 3.8	12	4.0 - 24
Eastern Mediterranean	4.0	2.8 - 5.4	16	2.2 - 41
Europe*	18	16 - 19	54	47 - 61
South-East Asia	2.6	2.0 - 3.4	14	7.7 - 23
Western Pacific	4.6	3.5 - 5.9	16	7.4 - 28
Global	3.4	2.5 - 4.4	18	7.6 - 31

Source: Adapted from the WHO Global TB Report, 2018

*Region with the highest incidence of MDR/RR-TB globally

% = percentage

2.2. The African epidemic

Although WHO estimates that half a million new cases of MDR/RR-TB occurred worldwide in 2018, information on the true burden of the disease in the WHO African Region is limited and is likely under-estimated due to widespread lack of laboratory infrastructure, poor surveillance mechanisms and lack of financial resources to conduct drug resistance testing in many countries [1,2,26,27]. This situation has led to a great deal of missing data on MDR/RR-TB from this region. For instance, there is no national drug resistance survey (DRS) data from many countries including Angola, Burundi, Chad, Congo, Gabon, Guinea, Guinea-Bissau, Liberia, Libya, Mali, Mauritania and Niger (Figure 1; Figure 2; and Figure 3 above). However, national DRS were underway in five countries namely the Republic of Angola, Burundi, Chad, Guinea and Mali between 2018 and 2019 [1,2] (Figure 1 above).

Recent studies in South Africa [28] as well as in Ethiopia [26] report an increasing prevalence of DR-TB in SSA and the report of very large numbers of MDR-TB and extensively DR-TB (XDR-TB) cases in Tugela Ferry, South Africa in 2012 likely represents unrecognized and continent-wide epidemic [1,26,29]. In contrast, a systematic review and meta-analysis conducted by Musa et al. reported low levels of MDR-TB in SSA region estimated to be 2.1% (95% CI; 1.7-2.5%) among new TB cases [30]. However, latest surveillance data based on continuous surveillance system of routinely performed DSTs and national DRS collected by the Global TB Project in 2018 reported that Angola, Democratic Republic of Congo, Ethiopia, Kenya, Mozambique, Nigeria, Somalia, South Africa and Zimbabwe accounted for the highest burden of MDR/RR-TB in the African WHO Region and are among the 27 high MDR/RR-TB burden countries in the world [1,2]. MDR/RR-TB cases among new cases in these countries ranged from as low as 1.7% in the Democratic Republic of Congo to as high as 8.7% in Somalia and among previously treated TB cases ranged from 4.4% in Kenya to as high as 47% in Somalia [1] (Table 2).

Sub-Saharan Africa	Percentage of new cases with MDR /RR-TB	Range	Percentage of previously treated cases with MDR/RR-TB	Range
Angola	2.4	1.1 – 4.2	15	11 - 19
DR Congo	1.7	1.1 – 2.6	9.5	8.8 - 10
Ethiopia	0.71	0.62 – 0.8	16	14 - 17
Kenya	1.3	0.74 – 2	4.4	3.7 – 5.2
Mozambique	3.7	2.5 - 5.2	20	5.2 - 40
Nigeria	4.3	3.2 - 5.5	15	11 - 19
Somalia	8.7	6.1 – 12	47	29 - 65
South Africa	3.4	2.5 - 4.3	7.1	4.8 – 9.5
Zimbabwe	3.9	3.5 – 4.3	14	8.9 - 20

Table 2: Estimated incidence of MDR/RR-TB for high MDR-TB burden WHO African countries in 2018

2.3. Summary

The prevalence of resistance to commonly used anti-TB drugs is increasing worldwide and threatens to undermine effective global TB control. Although significant regional variability in the distribution of MDR/RR-TB has been recorded, every region and country of the world has reported increasing drug resistance. While in Africa the true burden of MDR/RR-TB is likely underestimated due to lack of resources to perform DRS. China, India and Russia are reported to have the highest burden MDR/RR-TB accounting for more than 50% of the world's total cases.

3. Diagnosis of MDR/RR-TB: Current tools and challenges

Definitive diagnosis of MDR/RR-TB requires that MTB be detected and resistance to anti-TB drugs determined. This can be accomplished by isolating the MTB by culture, identifying it as belonging to the MTB complex and conducting DST using solid or liquid media or by performing a WHO-endorsed molecular test to detect TB deoxyribonucleic acid (DNA) and mutations associated with drug resistance [1,23]. Thus, using standardized and reliable methods for diagnosing MDR- TB or RR-TB provides guidance to clinicians on the most appropriate and effective treatment regimen for patient management and global control of the disease [1,2,13]. Therefore, in this review, we describe the currently available WHO-recommended diagnostic tools for the diagnosis of MDR/RR-TB and highlight major challenges associated with their implementation in low- and middle- income countries.

3.1 WHO approved tools for diagnosing MDR/RR-TB

There are essentially two different startegies to diagnose MDR/RR-TB. These include phenotypic methods which involve culturing of MTB on solid or liquid media containing a specific antibiotic, or genotypic methods which target specific molecular mutations associated with resistance against individual anti-TB drugs [1,14,24]. Both phenotypic and genotypic methods are suitable for use at different levels of the tiered network of TB laboratories for clinical management of patients and public health [14,17,24] and may be performed as a direct test (i.e. inoculation of media with the decontaminated sputum specimen) or as an indirect test (i.e. inoculation of media with a pure growth from a primary culture) [23,31-33].

3.1.1. Phenotypic (conventional) methods

Traditionally, these include culture-based methods [34]. Various techniques are available and are based on assessing the ability of MTB to grow in culture media containing a critical concentration of specific anti-TB agents (which indicates resistance) or conversely, its inability to grow in the same media (which indicates susceptibility) [14,35,36]. Thus, the standard conventional culture-based DST using Löwenstein-Jensen Proportion Method (LJPM), include the proportion method, the absolute concentration method and the resistant ratio method and the results obtained among the three methods for first-line anti-TB drugs do not differ significantly. However, the proportion method remains the most preferred choice for DSTs in low- and middle- income countries [14,34,36].

3.1.1.1. Proportion method

The indirect LJPM is the most common conventional culture-based method for testing the susceptibility of MTB isolates in resource limited settings (RLS) [14,34,36]. In order to perform phenotypic DST using this method, *mycobacteria* are initially grown on solid media and bacterial growth is identified macroscopically (i.e. by identifying specific characteristics of the colonies). The colonies identified are then typed to confirm the detection of MTB complex and to exclude the presence of any non-tuberculous mycobacteria or other bacteria prior to performing a DST [14]. Drug resistance is performed by inoculating the drug containing media with a defined inoculum of MTB and dilutions of the inoculum are also used to inoculate the drug-free control medium. The growth (i.e. the number of colonies) on a control medium without an anti-TB agent is compared with the growth present on a medium containing critical concentration of anti-TB agent being tested. Resistance is defined when at least 1% of growth is observed in drug-containing culture medium [14].

This traditional method is simple, reliable, easily accessible and cost-effective. However, the major challenge with conventional DST method is that results are only available after 4-8 weeks following standard culture. This diagnostic delay may lead to patients being inappropriately treated, drug resistance strains may continue to spread to uninfected individuals, and resistance may become amplified leading to increased morbidity and mortality [9,37]. Another challenge associated with this method is the requirement for sophisticated biosafety facilities that are expensive to build and maintain [15,21,38]. Furthermore, the use of this technique is only limited to national or central reference laboratory level or regional level laboratories which have appropriate infrastructure, equipment and adequate staff skills [38].

3.1.1.2. Liquid culture-based methods

The commercial liquid culture systems are the most modern and rapid phenotypic method for performing DST. These systems have been thoroughly evaluated in clinical settings and have been endorsed by WHO and Centers for Disease Control and Prevention (CDC) for rapid detection of TB drug resistance [38-40]. The commercial liquid culture systems available include MB/Bact (Biomerieux), Bactec 9000 (Becton Dickinson), ESPII (TREK Diagnostic systems, Inc) and the Bactec MGIT 960 system (Becton Dickinson, USA) [41]. The latter is rapidly becoming the method of choice in high throughput settings of low- and middle-income countries and is available as a manual and automated technique [36,42].

The Bactec MGIT 960 system is a non-radiometric system that uses a modified Middlebrook 7H9 broth combined with fluorescence quenching-based oxygen sensor to detect bacterial growth. The indicator fluoresces under ultra-violet (UV) light following the oxygen reduction induced by aerobically metabolizing mycobacteria within the medium. All positive cultures are typed to confirm the detection of MTB complex and to exclude the presence of any non-tuberculous mycobacteria or other bacteria prior to performing a DST [14]. DST is conducted using four anti-TB drugs: INH, RIF, SM, and EMB. To each 7 ml MGIT tube, 0.8 ml of MGIT 960 growth supplement, 0.1 ml of the drug stock solution and 0.5 ml of the test inoculum are added. For each isolate, a growth control (GC) tube with growth supplement and without a drug is included. All the inoculated tubes including one drug-free tube for each isolate are placed into the Bactec MGIT 960 instrument on the same day of inoculation. During incubation in the MGIT instrument, the fluorescence of drug-containing tubes is compared with that of the drug-free GC. The ratio of the relative growth of the drug-containing tube and that of the GC tube is determined by the system's software algorithms. If the relative growth in the drug-containing tube is equal to or exceeded that of the GC tube, the isolate is considered drug resistant; if the relative growth is less than that in the GC tube, the isolate was considered drug susceptible [36].

Several published studies have demonstrated excellent performance of the Bactec MGIT 960 system over the conventional culture-based DST for the rapid detection of resistance to first-line anti-TB drugs with very high sensitivity and specificity of nearly 100 % [41,42]. The average time to DST results with Bactec MGIT 960 system is two to four weeks compared with the 28-42 days needed for DST using the conventional DST [24,38,42-44]. However, Bactec MGIT 960 system like any other liquid culture systems come with a number of challenges: firstly, the assay is prone to contamination by other non-mycobacterial organisms or non-tuberculous mycobacteria [45,46,47]; secondly, the high cost of equipment and consumables of this technique compared with the conventional culture-based DST method hamper widespread implementation of this technology in low- and middle-income countries [24,47]; thirdly, liquid culture systems for DST require sophisticated laboratory infrastructure, higher biosafety facilities and high maintenance cost of the equipment [38].

3.1.1.3. New rapid phenotypic methods

New rapid non-commercial phenotypic methods for TB drug resistance have become available in the recent past and are recommended by WHO for use in RLS that lack access to more sophisticated laboratory infrastructure and techniques. Among these methods are the microscopic observation drug susceptibility (MODS) assay, Nitrate reductase assay (NRA; Griess method), TK medium (Salubris Inc, MA, USA), FASTPlaque-Response bacteriophage assay (Biotec Laboratories Ltd, UK), Thin Layer Agar (TLA) method and the Colorimetric redox Indicator (CRI) methods [23,24,32,48]. These assays were recently assessed by WHO and were found to be faster compared to conventional culture-based DST in the detection of drug resistance [49]. The following sections describe the currently available new rapid phenotypic methods for the detection of MDR/RR-TB in low- and middle- income countries.

3.1.1.3.1. Microscopic observation drug susceptibility assay (MODS)

MODS assay is a rapid liquid culture-based technique for detection of MDR/RR-TB directly in sputum specimen. The assay uses an inverted light microscope to detect microscopic colonies of MTB grown in culture medium contained in sealed multiwell plastic plates and the organism is identified based on its distinctive morphology such as cording, strings or tangles [24,36]. This low-technology assay relies on three basic principles: first, that MTB grows faster in the liquid medium than in solid medium; second, that characteristic cord formation can be visualized microscopically in liquid medium at an early age; and third, that, the incorporation of anti-TB drugs from the onset permits rapid and direct DST testing of both INH and RIF concomitantly with the detection of bacterial growth [24,32,50].

Sputum specimens previously digested, decontaminated and concentrated are inoculated into drug-free and drug-containing media, followed by incubation. Growth in drug-free media indicates a positive culture, while growth in both drug-free and drug-containing media indicates resistance [24,32,50]. This technique is relatively inexpensive to perform compared to commercial broth-based liquid systems such as the Bactec MGIT 960. For the detection of MTB in sputum, MODS has been demonstrated in multicenter studies to be more sensitive and faster than automated liquid culture systems and solid culture-based methods (7, 13, and 26 days, respectively) [36,38]. Because MODS utilizes direct DST, the average TAT for the detection of MDR/RR-TB is also 7 days [24,32,38]. However, the requirement for biosafety level-3 facilities, trained and skilled laboratory staff and an inverted microscope poses a serious challenge in the implementation of this technology in many RLS [32,36,38,51,52]. Furthermore, the assay is not recommended for decentralization to lower level laboratories [24].

3.1.1.3.2. Nitrate Reductase Assay (NRA)

The NRA is a liquid or solid culture technique for the rapid detection of INH and RIF resistance in MTB [36]. The principle underlying this technique is based on the ability of actively growing MTB to reduce nitrate incorporated in the medium to nitrite which is detected by colour change in the medium following the addition of the Griess reagent [38,48,50]. Resistance testing is done by inoculating and incubating drug-free and drug-containing LJ media at 37°C for 7, 10, or 14 days. The detection of the pink-purple coloured reaction on both drug-free and drug-containing media following the addition of Griess reagent indicates resistance, while susceptible strains loose this capacity as they are inhibited by the antibiotic, leaving the medium colourless [48,50].

NRA assay is simple and inexpensive to perform and has been found to have comparable sensitivity and specificity with the conventional DST for the detection of INH and RIF resistance [38]. For a direct NRA the average TAT to DST results is approximately 14-21 days whereas for an indirect NRA it is between 5-12 days after obtaining a culture [48,53]. The major challenge with this method is the requirement for trained and skilled laboratory staff, and the need for specialized biosafety facilities which are expensive to build and maintain [23,38,41].

3.1.1.3.3. TK medium

TK medium (Salubris, Inc., MA, USA) is a novel colorimetric system that has been adapted for the rapid detection of drug resistance directly from sputum samples [24,51]. This colorimetric system indicates growth of MTB by the colour change in the growth medium usually as a result of its metabolic activity which enables an early and positive identification before bacterial colonies appear. TK medium also permits susceptibility testing for drug resistance, and allow for differentiation between MTB and non-tuberculous mycobacteria. The average TAT to obtain DST results with this method is estimated to be 11 days compared with 4-8 weeks required for conventional DST [24,51]. However, there is insufficient published evidence on the diagnostic accuracy and field performance of this tool in developing countries [24].

3.1.1.3.4. Mycobacteriophage-based assays

Mycobacteriophage-based tests have been evaluated for diagnosis of TB as well as DST. This technology uses bacteriophages to infect live MTB and detect the presence of viable MTB in clinical specimens as well as culture isolates [24,38]. Two methods have been developed in recent years: In the first method, the underlying principle is amplification of phages after their infection of MTB, followed by detection of progeny phages using sensor bacteria and measuring plaque formation. In the second method, the principle of the assay is based on the detection of light (using luminometry or photography) produced by luciferase reporter phages (LRP) after their infection of live MTB [24,36,54,55].

Currently, there is one commercial phage-based test on the market i.e. the FASTPlaque-TB® assay (Biotec Laboratories Limited, Ipswich, Suffolk, UK). The first generation test for detection of RIF resistance, the FASTPlaque-MDRi®, previously named FASTPlaque-RIF® were designed to detect RIF resistance in culture isolates, i.e. indirect testing. A new version of this kit, FASTPlaque-Response® has been developed for detection of drug resistance directly from sputum specimens [24,38,55]. Drug resistance is diagnosed when MTB is detected in samples that contain the drug (e.g. RIF), and when phage-based assays do not detect MTB in drug-containing samples, the strains are classified as drug sensitive [38,54,55].

A recent meta-analysis of the accuracy of phage-based methods (amplification as well as luciferase phage assays) for detecting RIF resistance in MTB concluded that these assays when performed with MTB culture isolates have a high sensitivity, but variable and slightly lower specificity [24]. In general phase-based assays are easy to perform and the time to diagnosis of TB and associated drug resistance is about 2-3 days [41]. However, the major challenges with this assay is luck of sufficient evidence available on their accuracy when performed directly on sputum samples and the requirement for a sophisticated laboratory infrastructure [24,46].

3.1.1.3.5. Thin Layer Agar (TLA) Assay

The TLA is a rapid non-commercial solid culture-based method designed to simultaneously detect growth of MTB colonies and indicate INH and RIF resistance directly from processed smear-positive sputum specimens [36,38]. This assay is inexpensive and a rapid alternative to conventional methods for DST of MTB. In this assay, quadrant petri dishes containing a thin layer of supplemented Middlebrook 7H10 or 7H11 agar are used. This quadrant petridish has four compartments with one being a drug-free GC, another containing para-nitrobenzoic acid (PNB), as a specific inhibitor of MTB complex; drugs INH and RIF in the 3rd and 4th quadrants respectively [36].

Drug resistance is performed by inoculating the TLA plate with sputum specimen, and incubated at 37°C in a 5% carbon dioxide incubator. Plates are read every 2 days and over a period of 4 weeks using a conventional microscope at 100X magnification. MTB microcolonies can be detected using a standard light microscope in as little as 7 days, with results for DST between 10 and 15 days [36,38]. Inhibition of growth in the compartment containing PNB while growing in drug-free GC media is considered positive for MTB complex. Resistance is defined as growth in the compartments containing RIF and INH [41].

Although faster than the conventional DST using LJPM and relatively inexpensive compared to other culture-based methods, the TLA technique is not as fast or as sensitive as the liquid culture system. However, the specificity and predictive values for INH and RIF resistance have been reported to be 100%, suggesting that this assay would be a favorable alternative when liquid culture systems are not available. As with the MODS assay, BSL-2 (and possibly BSL-3) facilities are required for testing, and the safe disposal of biohazardous material is needed [36,38]. A high contamination rate experienced with this method and a long TAT to obtain DST results pose a serious challenge in the implementation of this method in routine clinical practice [38].

3.1.1.3.6. Colorimetric redox indicator (CRI) method

CRI methods are non-commercial culture and DST methods that may represent a good alternative for the rapid detection of drug resistance in laboratories with limited resources [24]. These indirect methods are based on the reduction of a coloured indicator added to a liquid culture medium in a microtiter plate after MTB has been exposed in vitro to different antibiotics and different drug concentrations. The most common growth indicators used to perform this assay are: Alamar blue, 3-[4,5-dimethylthiazole-2-yl]-2,5-diphenyl tetrazolium bromide (MTT) and Resazurin. Resistance is detected in approximately 3-5 weeks and is indicated by a colour change in the indicator, which is proportional to the number of viable mycobacteria [23].

Several methods have been developed in the recent past and results of a recent systematic review and meta-analysis on the performance and diagnostic accuracy of

CRI methods on culture isolates found that the techniques are highly sensitive (pooled estimate 98%; 95CI 96% - 99%) and specific (pooled estimate 99%; 95CI 99% - 100%) for the detection of RIF resistance as well as INH resistance (pooled sensitivity 97%; 95CI 96% - 98%; pooled specificity 98%; 95CI 97% - 99%) [24,54]. These methods have also shown to be inexpensive to perform and have similar biosafety requirements as conventional culture-based DST [23]. However, major challenges associated with CRI methods include the long TAT to obtain DST results; tests cannot be performed directly on clinical specimens; and the assays are not recommended for decentralization to lower level laboratories [24,54].

3.1.2. Genotypic (Molecular) methods

Genotypic (molecular) assays have been developed in recent years as a result of limitations of conventional culture-based DST methods. These methods have revolutionized the diagnosis of MDR-TB and generally use polymerase chain reaction (PCR) techniques to detect the genetic mutations that are known to confer resistance to drugs [14,16]. Compared with phenotypic methods, genotypic assays have considerable advantages for programmatic management of DR-TB, in particular with regard to their speed, the standardization of testing, their potentially high throughput and the reduced requirements for laboratory biosafety [14,34]. Line probe assays (LPAs) and Xpert MTB/RIF assays are the current WHO-recommended and widely used genotypic assays in low- and middle- income countries [36,57,58].

3.1.2.1. Line Probe Assays

LPA are a family of novel DNA strip-based tests that use PCR and reverse hybridization methods for the rapid detection of MTB and drug resistance from pulmonary smear-positive specimens or culture isolates grown by conventional methods. This high throughput molecular genetic assay comprises three steps: DNA extraction, multiplex PCR amplification and reverse hybridization [57,58]. Currently, two LPAs are commercially available: the INNO-LiPA® Rif.TB kit (Innogenetics, Ghent, Belgium) and the GenoType® MTBDR assay (Hain Lifescience, Nehren, Germany). The INNO-LiPA® Rif TB assay has been developed for the rapid detection of MTB and RIF resistance [36,57,58]. A recent review and meta-analysis summarized the results obtained for the INNO-LiPA® Rif. TB test, and showed that this assay has high sensitivity and specificity when culture isolates are used. The majority of studies had sensitivities of 95% or greater, and nearly all were 100% specific [24,36]. However, the results are less accurate when the test is directly applied to clinical specimens such as sputum [24,57,58].

The GenoType® MTBDR assay developed in 2004 is a novel kit-based method designed to detect resistance to both RIF and INH simulteneously. This is accomplished by identification of mutations in the *rpo*B gene that confers resistance to RIF as well as mutations in the *kat*G gene for high-level INH resistance either in culture isolates or clinical specimens. The sensitivities of this assay was 99% for *rpo*B and between 70% and 90% for codon 315 of *kat*G associated mutations, with a specificity of 100% for both genes [24,36]. In order to improve the sensitivity of GenoType MTBDR assay, an advanced version of this assay, the GenoType MTBDR*plus* assay, that covers more mutations has been developed in recent years [36,57,58]. This assay targets the mutations included in the first generation assay and includes a broader selection of probes for the wild-type *rpo*B gene and mutations in the promoter region of *inhA* gene [24,36,57-59].

The GenoType MTBDR*plus* assay was evaluated with smear-positive specimens in a high volume diagnostic setting in South Africa and was found to have sensitivities of approximately 98.9% for the detection of RIF resistance, 94.7% for the detection of INH resistance, and 98.8% for the detection of MDR-TB [36]. In a meta-analysis, the pooled sensitivity and specificity for the GenoType MTBDR*plus* assay were 98.4% and 98.9%, respectively [36]. The TAT for this molecular LPA was short between 8 hours and 48 hours compared with 4-8 weeks required to produce DST results using conventional culture-based DST [20,57,60].

However, the complexity of testing using LPAs in RLS restricts the use of this technology to central reference laboratory level or regional level laboratories where appropriate infrastructure and biosafety precautions can be assured (i.e. use of three separate rooms for extraction, amplification and post amplification proceedures) [14,61]. The high cost of technology and reagents in addition to the requirement of well-trained and skilled laboratory staff have also hampered the wide applicability of these assays in RL/HBC where the need is greatest. Furthermore, the WHO and Stop TB Partnership does not recommend using this technique directly with smear-negative clinical specimens or sputum specimens with very low bacillary load in view of their limited sensitivity [14,38,52,60,62].

3.1.2.2. Xpert MTB/RIF assay

Xpert MTB/RIF assay (Cepheid, Sunnyvale, CA, USA) is a fully automated novel R-T PCR-based assay for rapid and simultaneous detection of MTB and resistance to RIF (reliable marker for MDR-TB) directly in clinical specimens [2,17,61,63]. Endorsed by WHO in December, 2010 and approved by the USA Food and Drug Administration (FDA) in 2013, the assay has been extensively evaluated in various geographical settings demonstrating its potential for rapid and accurate detection of drug resistance in RLS [23,61]. This molecular assay is unique in that it has simplified the process of molecular testing, fully integrating sample preparation, amplification and detection required for R-T PCR in a self-contained cartridge [56,59]. Xpert MTB/RIF assay has been found to have similar sensitivity, specificity and accuracy as conventional culture-based DST and has been strongly recommended by WHO as the initial diagnostic test among persons at risk of MDR/RR-TB or HIV associated TB [1,23,61,63,64].

The advantages of using Xpert MTB/RIF over the conventional culture-based DST, commercial liquid culture systems or LPAs for the detection of drug resistance is that the assay can be performed directly on clinical specimens and provide results much faster (i.e. within 2 hours) which allows the patient to be offered prompt, appropriate and effective second-line treatment [59,65] which leads to decreased morbidity and mortality, improved patient outcomes, and interruption of further transmission of the disease to uninfected population [66]. Furthermore, Xpert MTB/RIF is suitable for use at all levels of the health care system as it does not require sophisticated laboratory infrastructure. However, their implementation in RLS may be hampered by a higher financial cost of the equipment and consumables [41,63], the requirement for a stable and uninterrupted power supply in a diagnostic facility [14,60,67], the high cost of instrument maintenance and calibration [41,68], the requirement for a good air conditioned laboratory [69], and the requirement for the expanded conventional DST involving INH, SM and EMB for confirmation of MDR-TB and for monitoring treatment response [65,70-73]. Table 3 provides a summary of the current WHO- recommended diagnostic options for MDR/RR-TB for low- and middle- income countries.

Table 3: SUMMARY OF WHO-RECOMMENDED DIAGNOSTIC OPTIONS FOR MDR/RR-TB AND ASSOCIATED CHALLENGES

Diagnostic platform	Test name	Turnaround time	Descriptions and comments	Challenges
Solid culture	Lowenstein–Jensen Proportion method (LJPM)	4–8 weeks	Egg-based medium, inexpensive.	Long TAT Requires biosafety facilities that are also expensive to maintain
	Middlebrook and Cohn 7H10		Agar based medium. Less prone to contamination than LJPM, but more expensive.	Long TAT and expensive
Automated liquid culture systems	MGIT 960 system	8 days with smear positive and 2–4 weeks with smear negative specimens	Liquid culture systems. Fully automated systems that use either fluorimetric or colorimetric detection.	High cost of equipment and reagents High cost of equipment maintenance
Non-commercial WHO endorsed culture and DST techniques	Microscopic observation drug susceptibility (MODS) assay	Direct test: 7 days Indirect test: 3–4 weeks	MODS is a manual liquid technique that uses basic laboratory equipment (including an inverted microscope). MTB colonies are observed through the bottom of a sealed plastic container and	Requirement for an inverted microscope Assay not recommended for decentralization to lower level laboratories

			allows for INH/RIF DST.	
	Nitrate reductase assay (NRA)	Direct NRA test: 14-21 days Indirect NRA test: 5–12 days after culture	NRA is a colorimetric test using solid media. Allows for INH/RIF DST. TB cells are cultured for 10 days and Greiss reagent is added, which indicates the presence of growing cells.	Long TAT Assay not recommended for decentralization to lower level laboratories
	Colorimetric redox indicator (CRI)	3–5 weeks	CRI is an indirect colorimetric test using liquid media. TB cell are cultured in the presence of a dye. Allows for INH and RIF DST.	Long TAT Assay not recommended for decentralization to lower level laboratories Lack of evidence on sensitivity and specificity of the assay
Genotypic (Molecular) testing	Line probe assay (LPA)	24–48 hours (direct on smear positive specimen only).	Strip test simultaneously detects TB genetic mutations for INH/RIF resistance. DNA targets are amplified by PCR	Requires 3 separate rooms High cost of reagents Requires trained and skilled laboratory

			and hybridized to immobilized oligonucleotide targets. Results are visualized calorimetrically.	personnel
	Xpert MTB/RIF	2 hours	A fully automated test for the detection of MTB and RIF resistance directly in clinical specimens, using real time PCR.	High cost of the diagnostic machines and reagents High cost of maintenance Requires stable and uninterrupted power supply Requires adequately trained laboratory staff

Adopted from Companion Handbook to the WHO Guidelines for the Programmatic Management of Drug-Resistant Tuberculosis. Geneva: WHO; 2014

4. Conclusion

Phenotypic and genotypic DST methods for MDR/RR-TB exist. However, the best strategy for the detection of MDR/RR-TB and the current WHO-recommended strategy, is to use novel rapid genotypic methods which allow for early detection of drug resistance and prompt initiation of appropriate and effective treatment with the potential for improved patient outcomes, reduced morbidity and mortality, and interruption of further transmission of the disease to uninfected population. However, cost of equipment and reagents as well as staff skills hinders the implementation of these technologies in RLS. Therefore, in an effort to effectively diagnose MDR/RR-TB, support from governments and international funding agencies such as WHO, Stop TB partnership, Global Fund and FIND in the development and implementation of novel rapid genotypic assays such as LPA, Xpert MTB/RIF and other simple, low cost molecular assays in low- and middle- income countries is essential and urgently needed.

5. Recommendations

Based on this review, the following constitutes the recommendations for low- and middle-income countries for widespread implementation of WHO-recommended diagnostic options in light of the recent developments in global TB control:

1.   The use of existing WHO-recommended diagnostic techniques in low- and middle-income countries must be accelerated and their use fully optimized.

2.   MGIT 960 liquid culture and DST systems, LPAs and Xpert MTB/RIF assay are highly recommended for widespread use.

3.   Conventional DST capacity is still needed for expanded DST for anti-TB agents other than RIF and INH.

4.   Xpert MTB/RIF assay is suitable and recommended for use at all levels of the laboratory network.

5.   The selection of the DST method should consider the following key attributes: accuracy, cost of the test, shelf life of reagents, sensitivity and specifity of the assay, sample throughput, personnel skills, availability of instrument service and technical assistance as well as the TAT of the assay.

6.   Further research is required for the development of simple, cheap, accurate and rapid molecular assays for use in low-and middle-income countries that can simuteneously detect INH and RIF resistance directly in clinical specimens.

REFERENCES

1. World Health Organization. Global Tuberculosis Report 2019. Geneva: World Health Organization, 2019. WHO/CDS/TB/2019.11.

2. World Health Organization. Global Tuberculosis Report 2018. Geneva: World Health Organization, 2018. WHO/CDS/TB/2018.20.

3. Botswana Ministry of Health. National Tuberculosis Control Program Combined Annual Report 2013 - 2014. Ministry of Health, Republic of Botswana, Gaborone, pp22.

4. Taghizade MH, Emami MZ, Khademi GH, Bahreini A, Saeidi M. Tuberculosis: Past, Present and Future. *Int J Pediatr* 2016; 4(1): 1243-54.

5. Pandey P, Pant ND, Rijal KR, Shrestha B, Kattel S, Banjara MR, Maharjan B, Rajendra KC. Diagnostic Accuracy of GeneXpert MTB/RIF Assay in Comparison to Conventional Drug Susceptibility Testing Method for the Diagnosis of Multidrug-Resistant Tuberculosis. *PLoS ONE* 2017 12(1).

6. Nebenzahl-Guimaraes H, Verhagen LM, Borgdorff MW, van Soolingen D. Transmission and progression to disease of *Mycobacterium tuberculosis* Phylogenetic lineages in The Netherlands. *J Clin Microbiol*. 2015; 53:3264-3271.

7. Narasimhan P, Wood J, MacIntre CR, Mathai D. Risk Factors for Tuberculosis. *Pulm Med. 2013;* 2013: 828939.

8. Pawlowski A, Jansson M, Sköld M, Rottenburg ME, Källenius G. Tuberculosis and HIV. *PLoS Pathog*. 2012 Feb; 8(2).

9. Desissa F, Workineh T, Beyene T. Risk factors for the occurrence of multidrug-resistant tuberculosis among patients undergoing multidrug – resistant tuberculosis treatment in East Shoa, Ethiopia. *BMC Public Health* 2018 18:422.

10. Daniel O, Osman E. Prevalence and risk factors associated with drug resistant TB in South West Nigeria. *Asian Pac J Trop Med*. 2011 Feb; 4(2):148-51.

11. Girum T, Tariku Y, Dessu S. Survival Status and Treatment Outcome of Multidrug-Resistant Tuberculosis (MDR-TB) among Patients Treated in Treatment Initiation Centers (TIC) in South Ethiopia: A Retrospective Cohort Study. *Ann Med Health Sci Res*. 2017; 7:331-336.

12. World Health Organization. Global Tuberculosis Report 2017. Geneva: World Health Organization; 2017.

13. World Health Organization. Global Tuberculosis Report 2016. World Health Organization; 2016. WHO/HTM/TB/2016.13.

14. Gilpin C, Korobitsyn A, Weyer K. Current tools available for the diagnosis of drug-resistant tuberculosis. *Ther Adv Infect Dis*. 2016 Dec; 3(6): 145-151.

15. World Health Organization. Technical manual for drug susceptibility testing of medicines used in the treatment of tuberculosis. Geneva: World Health Organization; 2018. (WHO/CDS/TB/2018.24).

16. Seung KJ, Keshavjee S, Rich ML. Multidrug-Resistant Tuberculosis and Extensively Drug-Resistant Tuberculosis. *Cold Spring Harb Perspect Med*. 2015 Sep 5(9): a017863.

17. Drobniewski F, Nikolayevskyy V, Maxeiner H, Balabanova Y, Casali N, Kontsevaya I, Ignatyeva O. Rapid diagnostics of tuberculosis and drug resistance in the industrialized world: clinical and public health benefits and barriers to implementation. *BMC Medicine* 11, article number: 190 (2013).

18. Mibei DJ, Kiarie JW, Wairia A, Kamene M, Okumu ME. Treatment outcomes of drug-resistant tuberculosis patients in Kenya. *Int J Tuberc Lung Dis*. 2016; 20(11): 1477-1482.

19. Patel SV, Nimavat KB, Alpesh PB, Shukla LK, Shringarpure KS, Mehta KG, Joshi CC. Treatment outcome among cases of multidrug-resistant tuberculosis (MDR-TB) in Western India: A prospective study. *J Infect Public Health*. 2016 July-Aug; 9(4): 478-484.

20. Falzon D, Schünemann HJ, Harausz E, González-Angulo L, Lienhardt C, Jalamillo E, Weyer K. World Health Organization treatment guidelines for drug resistant tuberculosis, 2016 update. *Eur Resp J*. 2017; 49: 1602308.

21. Bwanga F, Hoffner S, Haile M, Joloba ML. Direct susceptibility testing for multidrug resistant tuberculosis: A meta-analysis. *BMC Infect Dis* 9, 67 (2009).

22. Franden G, Pennington SS. Abrams' Clinical Drug Therapy: Rationales for Nursing Practice. 10th Edition, pp351; Wolter Kluver Health and Lippincott Williams and Wilkins, 2014.

23. World Health Organization. Companion Handbook to the WHO Guidelines for the Programmatic Management of Drug-Resistant Tuberculosis. Geneva: World Health Organization; 2014.3, laboratory.

24. Migliori GB, Matteelli A, Cirillo D, Pai M. Diagnosis of multidrug-resistant tuberculosis and extensively drug-resistant tuberculosis: Current standards and challenges. *Can J Infect Dis Med Microbiol*. 2008 Mar; 19(2): 169-172.

25. Li X, Deng Y, Wang J, Jing H, Shu W, Qin J, Pang Y, Ma X. Rapid Diagnosis Of Multidrug-Resistant Tuberculosis Impacts Expenditures Prior To Appropriate Treatment: A Performance And Diagnostic Cost Analysis. *Infect and Drug Resist*. 2019; 12 pages 3549-3555.

26. Mulisa G, Workneh T, Hordofa N, Suaudi M, Abebe G, Jarso G. Multidrug-resistant *Mycobacterium tuberculosis* and associated risk factors in Oromia Region of Ethiopia. *Int J Infect Dis*. 2015 Oct; 35: 57- 61.

27. Zumla A, Petersen E, Nyirenda T, Chakaya J. Tackling the Tuberculosis Epidemic in sub-Saharan Africa – unique opportunities arising from the second European Developing Countries Clinical Trials Partnership (EDCTP) programme 2015-2024. *Int J Infect Dis. 2015Mar;* 32: 46-9.

28. Gandhi NR, Andrews JR, Brust JCM, Montreuil R, Weissman D, Heo M, Moll AP, Friedland GH, Shah NS. Risk Factors for Mortality among MDR- and XDR-TB Patients in a High HIV-Prevalence Setting. *Int J Tuberc Lung Dis*. 2012 Jan; 16(1): 90-97.

29. Botswana Ministry of Health. Botswana Tuberculosis and Leprosy Programme: Annual Report, 2012. Ministry of Health, Republic of Botswana, Gaborone pp1-14.

30. Musa BM, Adamu AL, Galadanci NA, Zubayr B, Odoh CN, Aliyu MH. Trends in prevalence of multidrug resistant tuberculosis in sub-Saharan Africa: A systematic review and meta-analysis. *PLoS ONE*. 2017; 12(9).

31. Parsons LM, Somoskovi A, Urbanczik R, Salfinger M. Laboratory diagnostic aspects of drug resistant tuberculosis. *Frontiers in Bioscience* 2004: 9, 2086-2105.

32. World Health Organization. Companion HandBook to the World Health Organization Guidelines for the Programmatic Management of Drug Resistance Tuberculosis. Geneva: World Health Organization; 2014.

33. Caminero JA, Cayla JA, García-García J-M, García-Pérez FJ, Palacios JJ, Ruiz-Manzano J. Diagnosis and Treatment of Drug – Resistant Tuberculosis. *Arch De Bronconeumol*. 2017; 53(9): 501-509.

34. Koch A, Cox H, Mizrahi V. Drug-resistant tuberculosis: challenges and opportunities for diagnosis and treatment. *Curr Opin in Pharmacol*. 2018 Oct; 42:7-15.

35. Aung WW, Ei PW, Nyunt WW, Swe TL, Lwin T, Htwe, MM, Kim KJ, Lee JS, Kim Ck, Cho SN, Song SD, Chang CL. Phenotypic and Genotypic Analysis of Anti-Tuberculosis Drug Resistance in *Mycobacterium tuberculosis* Isolates in Myanmar. *Ann Lab Med*. 2015 Sep; 35(5): 494-499.

36. Parsons LM, Somoskövi Á, Gutierrez C, Lee E, Paramasivan CN, Abimiku A, Spector S, Roscigno G, Nkengasong J. Laboratory Diagnosis of Tuberculosis in Resource-Poor Countries: Challenges and Opportunities. *Clin. Microbiol Rev*. Apr. 2011, p.314-350.

37. Auld AF, Agizew T, Pals S, Finlay A, Ndwapi N, Boyd R. Implementation of a programmatic, stepped-wedge cluster randomized trial to evaluate impact of Botswana' s Xpert MTB/RIF diagnostic algorithm on TB diagnostic sensitivity and early anti-retroviral therapy mortality. *BMC Infectious Diseases*. 2016 16:606.

38. Stop TB Partnership and World Health Organization. New Laboratory Diagnostic Tools for TB Control. Geneva, World Health Organization; 2008.

39. Ghiasi M, Pande T, Pai M. Advances in Tuberculosis Diagnostics. *Curr Trop Med Rep* **2,** 54–61 (2015).

40. Ahmad S, Mokaddas E, Al-Mutairi N, Eldeen HS, Mohammadi S. Discordance across Phenotypic and Molecular Methods for Drug Susceptibility Testing of Drug-Resistant Mycobacteria tuberculosis isolates in a low TB Incidence Country. *PLoS ONE* 2016 11(4).

41. Hoek KGP. Investigation into Genotypic Diagnostics for Mycobacterium tuberculosis. Published dissertation presented for the degree of Doctor of Philosophy (Medical Biochemistry) at University of Stellenbosch, December, 2010.

42. Koh WJ, Ko Y, Kim CK, Park KS, Lee NY. Rapid diagnosis of tuberculosis and multidrug resistance using a MGIT 960 system. *Ann Lab Med*. 2012 Jul; 32(4): 264-269.

43. Raizada N, Sachdeva KS, Chauhan DS, Malhotra B, Reddy K, Dave PV, Mundade Y, Patel P, Ramachandran R, Das R, Solanki R, Wares DF, Sahu S, O'Brien R, Paramasivan CN, Dewan PK. A Multi-Site Validation in India of the Line Probe Assay for the Rapid Diagnosis of Multidrug-Resistant Tuberculosis Directly from Sputum Specimens. *PLoS ONE* 2014 9(2).

44. Siddiqi S, Ahmed A, Asif S, Behera D, Javaid M, Jani J, et al. Direct Drug Susceptibility Testing of *Mycobacterium tuberculosis* for Rapid Detection of Multidrug Resistance using the BACTEC MGIT 960 SYSTEM: a multicenter study. *J Clin Microbiol.* 2012 Feb; 50(2): 435-440.

45. Mueller DH, Mwenge L, Muyoyeta M, Muvwimi MW, Tembwe R, Mc Nerney R, Faussett PG, Ayles HM. Costs and cost effectiveness of tuberculosis cultures using solid and liquid media in developing country. *Int J Tuberc Dis. 2008*; 12(10): 1196-1202.

46. Ashavaid T.F. (ed). Laboratory Medicine in India, An Issue of Clinics in Laboratory Medicine. Clin Lab med 32 (2012) XV-Xviii. W.B. Saunders, 2012 New York.

47. Lawson L, Emenyonu N, Abdurrahman ST, Lawson JO, Uzoewulu GN, Sogaolu OM, Ebisike JN, Parry CM, Yassin MA, Cuevas L. Comparison of *Mycobacterium tuberculosis* drug susceptibility using solid and liquid culture in Nigeria. *BMC Research notes* 6, article number: 215 (2015).

48. Affolabi D, Odoun M, Martin A, Palomino JC, Anagonou S, Portaels F. Evaluation of Direct Detection of *Mycobacteria Tuberculosis* Rifampicin Resistance by a Nitrate Reductase Assay Applied to Sputum Samples in Cotonou, Benin. *J Clin Microbiol*. July 2007, p. 2123-2125, Vol.45, No.7.

49. Hmama Z. Management of Drug Resistant Tuberculosis: Current issues in Diagnosis and Management. IntechOpen 2013.

50. Halwai D, Gurung R, Poudyal N, Baral D, Bhattacharya SK. Evaluation of nitrate reductase assay in 7H11 agar for diagnosis of multidrug-resistant tuberculosis in eastern Nepal. *Trop Med Health*. 2018;46:26.

51. Dash M. Drug resistant tuberculosis: A diagnostic challenge. *J Postgrad Med* 2013; 59:196-202.

52. Groessl EK, Ganiats TG, Hillery N, Trollip A, Jackson RL, Catanzaro DG, Rodwell TC, Garfein RS, Rodrigues C, Crudu V, Victor TC, Catanzaro, A. Cost analysis of rapid diagnostics for drug-resistant tuberculosis. *BMC Infectious Diseases* volume 18, Article number: 102 (2018).

53. Gupta A, Sen MR, Mohapatra TM, Anupurba S. Evaluation of the Performance of Nitrate Reductase Assay for Rapid Drug-susceptibility Testing of *Mycobacterium tuberculosis* in North India. *J Health Popul Nutr*. 2011 Feb; 29(1): 20-25.

54. World Health Organization. Noncommercial Culture and Drug-Susceptibility Testing Methods for Screening Patients at Risk for Multidrug-Resistant Tuberculosis: Policy Statement. Geneva: World Health Organization; 2011.

55. Minion J, Pai M. Bacteriophage assays for rifampicin resistance detection in mycobacterium tuberculosis: updated meta-analysis. *Int J Tuberc Lung Dis*. 2010; 14(8):941-951.

56. PangY, Dong H, Tan Y, Deng Y, Cai X, Jing H, Xia H, Li Q, Ou X, Su B, Li X, Zhang Z, Li J, Zhang J, Haun S, Zhao Y. Rapid diagnosis of MDR and XDR tuberculosis with the MeltPro TB assay in China. *Scientific Reports* **6,** Article number: 25330 (2016).

57. Nguyen TNA, Anton-Le Berre V, Baňuls A-L, Nguyen TVA. Molecular Diagnosis of Drug-Resistant Tuberculosis: A Literature Review. *Front. Microbiol.* 10:794.

58. Ling DI, Zwerling AA, Pai M. Rapid diagnosis of drug resistant TB using Line probe assay: from evidence to policy. *Expert Rev. Resp. Med.* 2(5), 583-588 (2008).

59. Lacoma A, Garcia-Sierra N, Prat C, Ruiz-Manzano J, Haba L, Rosés S, Maldonado J, Domínguez J. GenoType MTBDR*plus* Assay for Molecular Detection of Rifampicin and Isoniazid Resistance in Mycobacterium Tuberculosis Strains and Clinical Samples. *J. Clin Microbiol.* Nov. 2008 p. 3660-3667.

60. Laniado-Laborín R. Clinical challenges in the era of multiple and extensively drug-resistant tuberculosis. *Rev Panam Salud Publica*. 2017; 41:e167.

61. Zijenah LS. The Recommended TB Diagnostic Tools, Tuberculosis, Jean-Marie Ntumba Kayembe, IntechOpen, 2018; DOI:10.5772/Intechopen.73070.

62. Yadav RN, Singh BK, Sharma SK, Sharma R, Soneja M, Sreenivas V et al. Evaluation of GenoType MTBDR*plus* Line Probe Assay with Solid Culture Method in Early Diagnosis of Multidrug Resistant Tuberculosis (MDR-TB) at a Tertiary Care Centre in India. *PLoS ONE* 2013; 8(9): e72036.

63. Martin LJ, Roper M. H, Grandjean L, Gilman RH, Coronel J, Caviedes L, Friedland JS, Moore DAJ. Rationing tests for drug-resistant tuberculosis – who are we prepared to miss? *BMC Med* 14, 30(2016).

64. Shenai S. WHO recommended tools to improve diagnosis of active and drug resistant tuberculosis. *Acta Med Int* 2015; 2:118-29.

65. World Health Organization. Xpert MTB/RIF Implementation Manual. Technical and Operational "how-to": practical considerations. Geneva: World Health Organization; 2014.5 Testing and managing patients. WHO/HTM/TB/2014.1.

66. Falzon D, Jaramillo E, Schünemann HJ, Arentz M, Bauer M, Bayona J, Blanc L, Caminero JA et al. WHO guidelines for the programmatic management of drug-resistant tuberculosis: 2011 update. *ERJ Express* 2011.

67. Prasad R, Gupta N, Banka A. Multidrug-resistant tuberculosis/rifampicin-resistant tuberculosis: Principles of management. *Lung India*. 2018 Jan-Feb; 35 (1): 78-81.

68. Pantoja A, Fitzpatrick C, Vassall A, Weyer K, Floyd K. Xpert MTB/RIF for diagnosis of tuberculosis and drug-resistant tuberculosis: a cost and affordable analysis. *Eur Respir J*. 2013; 42: 708-720.

69. Lawn SD, Mwaba P, Bates M, Piatek A, Alexander H, Marais BJ et al. Advances in tuberculosis diagnostics: the Xpert MTB/RIF assay and future propects for a point-of-care test. *Lancet Infect Dis.* 2013 Apr; 13(4):349-361.

70. Shah M, Chihota V, Coetzee G, Churchyard G, Dorman SE. Comparison of laboratory costs of rapid molecular tests and conventional diagnostics for detection of tuberculosis and drug- resistant tuberculosis in South Africa. *BMC infect Dis* 2013 Jul 29; 13: 352.

71. Ardizzoni E, Mulders W, Kotrikadze T, Aspindzelashvili R, Goginashvili L, Pangtey H, Varaine F, Bastard M, Rigouts L, de Jong BC. The thin-layer agar method for direct phenotypic detection of multi- and extensively drug-resistant tuberculosis. *Int J Tuberc Lung Dis* 19(12):1547–1552.

72. World Health Organization. Implementing tuberculosis diagnostics: Policy framework. World Health Organization; 2015; WHO/HTM/TB/2015.11.

73. World Health Organization. Rapid implementation of the Xpert MTB/RIF diagnostic test: technical and operational "How-to" practical considerations. World Health Organization; 2011; WHO/HTM/TB/2011.2

About the authors

Dr. Blackson Pitolo Tembo is an accomplished public health specialist working as a consultant / researcher in Zambia. Prior to his current position, he worked for Zambia`s Ministry of Health as a Lecturer in medical microbiology at Ndola Central Hospital - School of Biomedical Sciences. He also worked as a Principal Medical Laboratory Technician with Botswana Ministry of Health at Deborah Retief Memorial Hospital, Kasane Primary Hospital and the National Tuberculosis Reference Laboratory. With over 32 years experience in medical laboratory work, Dr. Tembo has also served as a consultant with American Society for Microbiology in the roll-out and implementation of Xpert MTB/RIF diagnostic technology as well as the implementation of the TB External Quality Assurance Programme in Botswana. He is a well-known trainer in Xpert MTB/RIF technology and Fluorescent microscopy. His interest in TB research covers mainly the development of rapid molecular techniques for diagnosis of drug resistance tuberculosis.

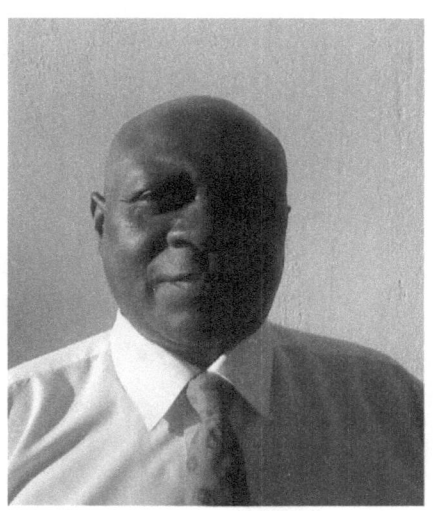

Professor Ntambwe Gustav Malangu was a pharmacoepidemiologist with public health expertise in drug safety issues. He worked in both private and public sectors of the healthcare industry in several African countries as an international health consultant and technical advisor. At the time of his death, he was the Head of Department of Epidemiology and Biostatistics at the School of Public Health of Sefako Makgatho Health Sciences University, Pretoria, South Africa. He was also the Production Editor for PULA: Botswana Journal for African Studies as well as a reviewer of international peer-reviewed journals.

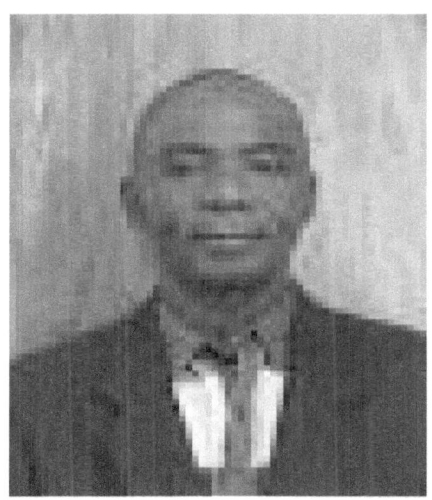